Beyond Weight Loss

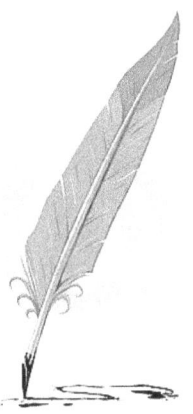

Raymond E. Smith

Published by
SanWay International
91 E. Main Street
Inman, SC 29349

Email: resco6042@yahoo.com
Website: www.SanwayInternational.com

Introduction

Why am I writing this book? Personally, I do not normally have a weight problem. There was one time in my life that I gained too much weight. I typically weigh about 160. In 1993, I gained up to 198. I was miserable. Fortunately, I knew how to get it off and I did. I lost it by controlling what I ate and I got a lot of natural exercise.

I learn to control what I ate by watching over-weight people grocery shopping. Over-weight people bought fattening foods. If you don't buy it – you can't eat it. By natural exercise I mean; fat people park close to the door of the store when going shopping, I parked at the other end of the parking lot. While waiting for my wife to go shopping I walked the circumference of the parking lot. When inside the store I walked up and down the aisles pushing the shopping cart. When visiting hospitals or a high-rise building I walked the stairs rather than take the elevator. A few common sense rules will take it off for most people, while others need further help. This book is going to cover all classes of weight-loss.

While over-weight I was miserable. It hurt to bend over and tie my shoes. I had problems with breathing. I was in construction and there were things I could not do because of the extra weight I was carrying. Thirty-eight pounds is not that much except it was all in my mid-section.

Beyond Weight Loss

More important than my own weight, my first wife gained 58 pounds with our first child and she never lost it. She had a saying that losing weight is no problem, because she had lost a ton. Unfortunately she regained what she lost and more. We called it the yo-yo syndrome. She weighted approximately 100 pounds when we married and when she died 44 years later she weight between 350 – 375 pounds. I never knew exactly what she weighted. She said, "I will tell you how old I am, but not how much I weigh." She became interested in losing weight when the doctor said she was obese. We will discuss this in a later chapter.

Regardless where you are today in regards to your weight this book will help you. I urge you to read it carefully. There are three main categories of things you need to consider if you have a weight problem; 1) What you eat, 2) exercise and 3) the right mental attitude. We will cover all three and more

Chapter One
Fad Diets

When considering a fad diet the name alone should tell you that it won't work. The best rule here is anything that is not a normal way of life will be very temporary. For instance; a total liquid diet is not a way of life because the body wants something to chew.

Fad diets may take it off for a short while, but you will put it back on and more with it. Let me say a word about the term diet. Your diet is what you eat. Everyone has a diet. The term has been taken completely out of context. Below are some fad diets that have come along in the past few years:

Acai Berry Diet: The acai berry has gained extreme popularity since being promoted on the Oprah Show. From my research the acai berry has some strong health benefits when used along with a balanced meal. To make a diet from it is a little too much. There are many foods discovered in the Amazons and the high mountains of India that are beneficial to our health when eaten with common sense.

Cabbage Soup Diet: This diet is not sustainable but continues to fall in and out favor.

HCG Diet: This diet has exploded in popularity in 2009, but

is it a legitimate way to lose weight or should the HCG diet be considered an unhealthy fad?

Hollywood diet: Low in Calories and involves drinking a "miracle juice".

Apple Cider Vinegar Diet Promotes using ACV to lose weight but too much can be harmful. Apple cider and vinegar are highly recommended for good health purposes when use in the proper amounts.

Sacred Heart Diet: Very low in calories and revolves around soup recipes.

Beverly Hills Diet: This diet supposedly reveals the rich celebrity's diet secrets.

Grapefruit Diet: This diet says that grapefruit burns fat, but grapefruit can interact with medication, so beware.

Tapeworm Diet: It is undeniable that people will resort to extreme measures in a desperate attempt to shed those extra pounds. But ingesting tapeworms in order to lose weight is not only a radical method but also an extremely dangerous one.

Atkins diet: Although written in the 1970s, Atkins Diet Revolution became a huge phenomenon only in the last few years.

Dukan Diet: This low carb diet came from France and shot to popularity.

Liquid Amino Diet: A low calorie diet combined with using amino acid/herb drops.

Low Fat diet: Very popular during the 1980s and 1990s.

Low Carb diet: Experienced a huge surge in popularity during 2003-2004 - but interest began to decline towards the end of 2004.

The 1 Day Diet: If You Know You Will Quit After 1 Day, Go With This One And Be A Success!

The 3 Day Diet: If You Think You Can Last For 3 Days, Here Is The Diet Plan For You.

Amputation Diet: If You Need To Lose Weight Fast At All Costs, Like To Win A Bet, Here Is The Plan For You. As I mentioned in the introduction my wife became interested in losing weight when the doctor told her she was obese. At that time obese was considered when one is 100 pounds over their ideal weight. Today they use the BMI to determine obesity.

How to determine your BMI:

Divide your weight in pounds by you height in inches squared. Multiply by 705. For example if a person is 5'6" and weighs 190 pounds:

Height of 5'6" = 66 inches. 66 squared is 66 x 66 = 4,356. 190 divided by 4,356 = 0.0436. 0.0436 x 705 = 30.75. This would be rounded off at 31.

BMI is categorized as follows:

Less than 18.5 – under weight

18.5 to 24.9 – normal weight

25 to 29.9 – over weight with health concerns

30 or more – obese

40 or more – morbid obese

She talked with her doctor about the best way to lose. It just happened that he was in the business of promoting stomach stapling. He talked her into doing the placation surgery. That is when they staple part of the stomach so you feel full sooner. When she left the hospital he gave her a shot glass and said you can eat this much three times a day for the next two months. As you know one cannot put much food into a shot glass. But, it matters what foods you put into the glass. A couple weeks after coming home she decided to eat some one of her favorite foods; macaroni. The macaroni started expanding in her stomach and it swelled more than the size of her stomach. When her stomach started swelling and the incision that was stapled opened and started losing a lot of blood. During her stay in the hospital I heard many scary stories about placation surgery. Some of it was due to stupidity. One lady decided she would eat all she wanted to eat to prove whether or not the staples would hold. She learned the hard way that there is a limit to the amount of food she should eat.

My wife got serious about the program and lost 123 pounds. She weighed 246 when she decided to get the surgery done. She got upset when I told people that she was half the women she used to be. I learned right away that I was making a mistake and stopped. After losing the weight and enjoying wearing smaller clothing and doing things she had not done in many years, the fad lasted about two months. She regained the 123 pounds and more.

While she had lost the weight we worked with a diet company as field trainers. We traveled the entire southeast meeting mostly with doctors who had purchased a large supply of products; teaching them how to promote the products.

There was one interesting moment while at a large meeting in a hotel I could not find my wife. After asking several people if they had seen her I said, "I knew some day this would happen. If she kept losing weight she would disappear." At least it got a good laugh.

Beyond Weight Loss

Remember, if it's not a normal way of life it won't last. To lose weight you must be willing to make some lifestyle changes.

Chapter Two
Dangers of Obesity

The number of over-weight people in America is astounding. According to government statistics; Mississippi was the most obese state in the United States at the end of 2009, followed by Louisiana. In 33 states, at least one quarter of the population was obese and in 11 others, more than 30 percent of the population had a BMI of 30 or more. The rate has risen dramatically since 1991, when no state recorded obesity rates in excess of 20 percent of the population. The least obese states at the close of 2009 were Colorado and Washington, D.C., the only two remaining states to record an obesity rate of less than 20 percent.

Although obesity rates are rising across all ethnic groups, statistically, African Americans are the most

overweight group in America, followed by Hispanics, then whites. Black individuals are 51 percent more likely to be obese than their Caucasian counterparts, and Hispanics are 21 percent more likely. Native Americans and Alaskan natives have a 32.4 percent rate of obesity, while Asian Americans have the lowest rate, only 8.9 percent.

Thirty percent of children in 30 states were obese as of July 2009. Mississippi also had the most overweight children in the age group of 10 to 17, with 44.4 percent of their youngsters, almost half, being obese. According to the Trust for America's Health, the obesity rates of this age group across all states tripled since 1980.

In recent months the federal government has gotten involved to help curb the obesity rate. Limits on the serving size of sodas, the types of foods served at schools and various programs are being implemented.

Obesity... overweight... fat. No questions, it's one of this nation's worst and most costly health problems. But, can government, in its finest "we know what's best for you" tradition, use laws to bring about the thinning of America?

According to a recent Washington Post article, legislatures in at least 25 states are currently debating more than 140 bills aimed at curbing obesity.

New state laws currently under consideration would restrict the sale of soda and candy in public schools, require fast-food chains to post fat and sugar content directly on all menu boards, and even attempt to tax the fat away.

According to the Post, six bills proposed by New York State Assemblyman Felix Ortiz (D) would slap hefty taxes on not only fatty foods, "but also modern icons of sedentary living -- movie tickets, video games and DVD rentals." Ortiz estimates his tax laws would haul in over $50 million a year, which New York could use to fund public exercise and nutrition programs.

"We have focused on smoking; now it is about time we fight obesity," Ortiz told the Post.

Over 44 million Americans are now considered obese, with an associated increase in cases of serious and costly diseases, including diabetes, heart disease and kidney failure. As costs to health plans of obesity-driven illnesses soar, the success of anti-smoking legislation passed during the 1990s and the seatbelt laws of the 1970s have lawmakers thinking similar laws could help force Americans to push away from the table.

Obviously, civil libertarians and consumer rights groups do not like the idea of legislating eating behavior. "It's an individual responsibility issue," states Richard Berman, executive director of the Center for Consumer Freedom in the Post article. "If I'm going to shorten my own life by eating too much or being too sedentary, that may not be much different than shortening my life by riding a motorcycle without a helmet on."

On the other hand, Health and Human Services Secretary Tommy G. Thompson cites the $117 billion spent annually on obesity-related health care when he states, "If we're really interested in holding down medical costs and improving the health of citizens, we have to do something about obesity."

Some insurance industry officials have suggested charging obese persons higher premiums. HHS Secretary Thompson, however, cautioned that doing so could run afoul of federal anti-discrimination laws.

The most potentially contentious fat-fighting suggestion mentioned in the Post story came from Eric Topol, chief of cardiology at the Cleveland Clinic. Topol's suggestion would offer a federal income tax credit to slender people, while "the people ruining our health care economics [the obese] would pay the standard tax."

People who are able to be disciplined and lose weight should be rewarded," said Topol.

According to Centers for Disease Control (CDC) there are

232 million people in the U.S. and Canada who are over-weight or obese.

What is Obesity costing the USA?

There is a familiar phrase that some people use; "It's my body and I will do what I want to do with it, it's not hurting any-one but me." If you have ever said this you need to pay attention to the next few lines.

When the economy experiences a recession, America tends to gain weight. Processed and fast foods are less expensive than nutritious foods, and tighter budgets may result in families eating poorly in terms of health and weight maintenance. Lean times also impact rates of depression and stress, and a common response to these emotions for many people is to eat.

The nation's obesity takes a heavy toll on Medicaid and Medicare programs as it results in increased rates of mortality from all causes. As of February 2010, Medicare paid out an additional $1,723 per person for those with a BMI of 30 or higher, while Medicaid paid out an additional $1,021 per person.

Who is paying the cost for obesity? You and I are. Every tax payer in America is sharing the costs.

There is nothing more dangerous to your health than being overweight. Those love handles are, put simply, your Death Warrant. There's no surer of way destroying your manhood and shortening your life than those extra pounds around your mid-section.

Let's look at some physical dangers of obesity for men.

Estrogen: Extra fatty tissue increases aromatize levels, leading to extra Estrogen in the male body. This is deadly over time, leading to decreased testosterone. Estrogen is also highly suspected of playing a role in prostate cancer.

Bad Sex: Those extra pounds are correlated with bad sex. No guy wants a poor sex life but some do not want to admit that the spare tire is dragging down their performance in the bedroom.

Erectile Dysfunction and Impotence: Being overweight is also a strong predictor of erectile dysfunction.

Low Testosterone: Being overweight is also associated with decreased free and total testosterone.

Inflammation: Fat cells, or adipose tissue in the literature, churn out cytokines, raising inflammation throughout your body, which is bad for the heart and penis.

Metabolic Syndrome and Insulin Resistance: Increases a hormone called resistin that leads to, you guessed it, insulin resistance, a.k.a. Metabolic Syndrome. Metabolic Syndrome is the curse of Western Societies.

Prostate Cancer: Increased risk of prostate cancer and other cancers. Researchers recently discovered that one reason this occurs is that one of the lipase enzymes that the body uses on stored fat actually turns on cancer cells into aggressive thrives and growers. In other words, your spare tire literally feeds and fuels cancers, which explains why obesity and cancer so often go hand in hand.

Decreased Fertility: Greatly decreased Fertility. The decreased testosterone and extra fat in the area of your scrotum kill and injure your sperm.

Blood Clots and Stroke: Increase plasminogen activator inhibitor which increases clotting which leads to increased risk for stroke and heart attack.

Arteriosclerosis and Heart Disease: Increases IL-6 leading to augmented blood vessel inflammation which in turn leads to increased arteriosclerosis. Decreases an anti-inflammatory compound called adiponectin, which leads to increased levels of IL-6 and arterial inflammation.

Hypertension and Blood Pressure: Extra body fat increases a bodily chemical called angiogenesis that raises blood pressure, one of the key enemies of your sexual and circulatory life.

Dementia: Increased risk of dementia due to excess abdominal fat in midlife.

Apnea and Sleep Disorders: Increases your likelihood for apnea, the sleep disorder where air is temporarily cut off during sleep. Apnea is associated with many disorders and problems, not to mention the fact that you never feel rested!

These are a few of the physical dangers associated with obesity for men. The list could go on.

Millions of Americans and people worldwide are overweight or obese. Being overweight or obese puts you at risk for many health problems. The more body fat that you have and the more you weigh, the more likely you are to develop:

Coronary heart disease
High blood pressure
Type 2 diabetes
Gallstones
Breathing problems
Certain cancers

This list applies to anyone who is obese. Your weight is the result of many factors. These factors include environment, family history and genetics, metabolism (the way your body changes food and oxygen into energy), behavior or habits, and more.

This is a few factors that apply to obese children.

Cardiovascular Disease: Overweight children and teens are at a higher risk for heart damage and circulatory conditions such as high cholesterol or high blood pressure, warns the National Center for Chronic Disease Prevention and Health Promotion. Poor dietary and eating habits in childhood and the teen years often carry into adulthood, increasing risk of obesity-related health and physical conditions. These not only include high blood pressure, but also heart disease, narrowed or blocked arteries in a condition called atherosclerosis and damage to tissues and organs caused by inadequate oxygenation or blood flow.

Poor Stamina: Children and teens that are overweight or obese are unable to maintain strength and stamina during sports or activities that require physical exertion. Shortness of breath, weakened joints and poor lung and heart function may severely limit the intensity of physical activity children may otherwise enjoy. Extreme weight places additional stress on the skeletal system, including the knees, hips and lower spine, often causing pain and stiffness.

Poor Self-Esteem: A child or teen that is overweight or obese may have very poor self-esteem and lack confidence. Peer pressure is strong through school, and those who are overweight may struggle with depression, suggests the National Center for Chronic Disease and Health Promotion.

Type 2 Diabetes: Children are just as apt to develop pre-diabetic and diabetic conditions as older adults, according to the University of Michigan Health System. Nearly one in three kids is now considered overweight, leaving them at a higher risk for problems later in life, including insulin-resistant type 2 diabetes. Foods high in sugars and fats also increase calories consumed while lack of exercise creates a calorie imbalance, warns the National Center for Chronic Disease Prevention and Health Promotion. The imbalance leaves the body overworked and vulnerable to high levels of glucose. High levels of sugar or glucose in the blood place additional stress on the kidneys and may lead to a condition called hyperglycemia.

Chapter 3

Foods

According to one doctor, "It is not just what you eat that decides who you are, but also what your mother ate." Based on this there are some serious consequences to being obese and having children. Not only does it damage your life, but the lives of future generations. This causes one to give serious thoughts to the foods you eat.

The New England Journal of Medicine gave this report on foods that make us fat.

The extensive study used data for over 120,000 healthy men and women from previous studies to track their diet every four years from 1986 to 2006 to see how their lifestyle and what they ate affected their weight. The researchers found that within each period the average weight gain was a little over three pounds — which added up to a 17-pound total weight gain over the 20-year period.

What caused that weight gain? Topping the list of culprits are meat, sweetened drinks, fried foods, and any form of potatoes. The biggest cause of weight gain was eating french fries; every extra serving of fries eaten in a day was linked to a gain of more than three pounds, while eating an extra serving of potato chips led to 1.69 pounds. Other diet busters included refined grains (like white rice and white bread) and butter.

But the news wasn't all bad; the study also identified the foods that helped prevent weight gain. Read on for the list of foods that cause and prevent weight gain.

Worst food offenders (pounds gained for every additional serving per day over four years):

French fries (over three pounds)

Potato chips (1.69 pounds)

Potatoes (1.28 pounds)

Sugar-sweetened drinks (one pound)

Red meat (0.95 pounds)

Processed meats (0.93 pounds)

Best foods for your waistline (amount of weight gain prevented for every additional serving):

Yogurt (-0.82 pounds)

Nuts (-0.57 pounds)

Fruits (-0.49 pounds)

Whole grains (-0.37 pounds)

Vegetables (-0.22 pounds)

The results show us what everyone knows — eating junk food and starchy foods can be bad news for your waistline — but the data are useful for quantifying just how much that extra bag of chips can hurt you, as well as how making the switch to whole healthy foods can help. Ready to make those changes?

If you aren't sure about a serving size follow these guidelines:

The size of a deck of cards is about the same as a three ounce serving of cooked meat, poultry or fish.

A baseball is about the same size as a cup of milk, yogurt, or chopped fresh greens.

A computer mouse is about the size of a cup of cut fruit, vegetables or pasta.

A tennis ball is about the same size as a medium piece of fruit.

Your whole thumb is about the size of an ounce of cheese.

Your thumb tip is about a teaspoon size of margarine or butter.

I traveled for a while with the president of a weight-loss company. When going to a restaurant for breakfast for example, he made certain demands. A scenario goes like this: The waitress comes to the table and says, "What can I get you this morning?" He answers, "I would like two scrambled eggs with plain toast, provided you cook the eggs the way I want them." She says, "Sir we will be happy to cook them any way you want them." He continues, "Take a paper towel and wipe the grill clean, no grease whatsoever. Then cook my eggs on the clean grill." The days I was with him I never heard a complaint. They prepared his breakfast just the way he ordered it.

My point is when eating out you have the right to demand your food to be the way you want it prepared. Don't be bashful or timid about asking for what you want.

As I mentioned earlier, I followed fat people around in the grocery store to see what they were buying. They were filling their shopping carts with cakes, candies, soda drinks, and other fattening foods. Some say, "I bought sugar free." I am sure you have heard this warning before, just because the label says "sugar free" doesn't mean that it is low in calories.

Weight gain is largely caused by the amount and types of foods we eat. After losing the 38 pounds several years ago I maintained 165 for many years. Two years ago I was diagnosis with cancer of the bone marrow (Multiple Myeloma). I was hospitalized twice with pneumonia. My appetite hit the bottom. Within a short while I had lost 35 pounds. My weight is presently holding at 137 pounds.

I plan to use this again in a later chapter, but I would like to tell you a true story of an experience with attitude in weight control. By the way, I choose to use the term weight control because no one wants to lose anything. Weight-loss has some negative connotations.

I was hired by a so-called diet company in the early 80s. We held weekly meetings in various locations throughout the southeast. The meetings were held wherever the host chose to have them. On this occasion we meet in a restaurant that had a good salad bar. The rule was that we would only eat salad. I watched several ladies fill their salad plates so full that they arranged sticks of celery so they could stack more food on their plate. It reminded me of my grandpa building sides on his old truck so he could haul more. After eating one of the ladies said, "You see, I told you I don't eat much. She was obviously very much overweight. While we are on the subject of eating salads, it's not always the amount of salad fixings; it's the dressing that gets you.

Bread

From what we are hearing today bread or wheat products may be the number one culprit for weight gain. According to the experts in my research during the 1980s the government started pushing the idea that Americans are not getting enough whole grain foods. The food manufactures jumped on the band wagon and started making more foods with whole grain and by doing so they increased the amount of flour consumed by the public.

Countless books and magazines are saying, "Stay away from wheat products and you will lose weight."

Prepackaged Meals:

Pre-packaged weight loss meals offer convenience and an easily accessible meal plan for people who want to lose weight. Americans spend more than $2 billion a year on pre-packaged frozen diet meals, according to Consumer Reports. With so many people purchasing frozen diet foods, it is helpful to examine what goes into pre-packaged diet foods, how they work and what the benefits and drawbacks are.

Features

There are a wide range of pre-packaged diet foods on the market, including an assortment of meal-replacement bars and shakes and boxed meals that are freshly prepared or frozen. Pre-packaged meals include a variety of vitamins and nutrients, and the boxed meals usually contain foods from at least a few of the food groups, such as grains, vegetables, meat and beans, fruit or milk. Freshly prepared boxed meals are usually available for pick-up or delivery to clients of specific weight loss services.

Benefits

Pre-packaged weight loss meals offer convenience and accessibility, helping dieters plan their eating without extensive calculations or nutrition research. Another benefit of pre-packaged diet meals is the quick preparation time for most meals, as they can require as little as unwrapping a snack bar to the few minutes required to cook a meal in the microwave. Pre-packaged meals also contain full nutrition information, making it easy to track your calories and daily nutrient intake.

Expert Insight

According to a Moores Cancer Center study reported in The Guardian article "Lasting Weight Loss Possible With Pre-Packaged Meals," it is possible to lose weight by eating pre-packaged diet meals, along with counseling and a structured weight loss program. In a trial with 442 overweight women, the subjects demonstrated that weight loss is possible with pre-made diet meals. Diet plans can offer help with nutritious eating, while an accompanying weight management program that incorporates healthy lifestyle habits and regular exercise will compliment the diet program.

Drawbacks

There may be some drawbacks to using a pre-packaged meal plan program to lose weight. Consumer Reports states that pre-packaged frozen foods can be high in sodium and have a bland taste. According to a Consumer Reports taste test of 24 diet en-trees, the taste of frozen meals has improved, as half of the meals were rated very well for taste. Some people do not like pre-packaged meals because of limited meal options or restricted choices of foods, although the food options can vary widely, de-

Beyond Weight Loss

pending on which program you choose.

Chapter 4

Recipes

The following recipes have been tried and proven for controlling your weight.

Broiler Chicken

3 chicken breast, split and skinned

2/3 cup low-calorie Italian dressing

¼ cup soy sauce

½ cup finely chopped onion

1 tsp dry mustard

Brush with sauce mixture. Place chicken in bottom of broiler pan. Broil 5 to 7 inches from heat for 20 minutes, brushing occasionally. Turn. Broil till meat is tender, about 20 minutes.

Serves 6 – 270 calories per serving.

Broiler Lemon Chicken

4 small boneless chicken breast

3 tbsp lemon juice

¼ cup slice green onions with tops

 1 tbsp water

1 tbsp salad oil

½ tsp dried crushed marjoram

¼ tsp granulated garlic

½ tsp dried crushed basil

¼ tsp dried crushed thyme

Dash seasoning salt

In a large zip-lock baggie place chicken and other ingredients. Marinate in baggie ½ hour at room temperature. Turn baggie frequently. Remove chicken from bag, reserving sauce and broil until done (approximately 25 minutes). Baste with marinate sauce as chicken broils, turning occasionally.

Serves 4 – 175 calories per serving.

Sautéed Chicken

1-1/2 pounds chicken

1 tbsp butter buds

1 tsp Worcestershire sauce

1 tsp garlic

1 large onion

1 cup fresh mushrooms

½ cup water

2 tsp cornstarch

1-1/2 bouillon cubes (chicken)

1 tbsp lemon juice

In skillet combine butter, Worcestershire sauce and garlic. Cook over medium heat until garlic is brown. Pour in mushrooms; add water, lemon juice and bouillon. Cover and simmer 25 minutes or until meat is done. Combine cornstarch and add ¼ cup cold water. Cook and stir until thickened and bubbly. Serve.

Serves 6 – 280 calories per serving.

Baked Flounder for Two

1 lb flounder fillets

1 cup mushrooms

¼ cup chicken bouillon broth

1 medium tomato, diced

2 tbsp parsley flakes

Garlic power to taste

Ground pepper to taste

Combine all ingredients except tomato. Place in baking dish and bake at 375 degrees for 15 to 20 minutes. Top each piece with ½ of the diced tomato.

Serves 2 – 205 calories per serving.

Scallops

2 tbsp butter buds

2 lbs scallops

2 tomatoes cut in ¼

¼ cup water

½ tbsp cornstarch

1 tsp soy sauce

½ tsp low sodium salt

¼ tsp pepper

Melt butter buds in a non-stick skillet. Add scallops and cook over low heat for 2 minutes. Add tomatoes. In bowl mix water, cornstarch, soy sauce, salt and pepper. Add mixture to skillet and cook until sauce is thick.

Serves 6 – 200 calories per serving.

Eggplant Parmesan

2 tbsp Italian seasoned breadcrumbs

2 tsp oregano

½ tsp granulated garlic

1 – 8oz can tomato sauce

3 – 1 oz slices low-fat mozzarella cheese

1 eggplant peeled and sliced thinly

2 tbsp grate parmesan cheese

Mix breadcrumbs, oregano, garlic and parmesan cheese. Soak eggplant for 5 minutes. Pat eggplant slices with a paper towel. Place eggplant slices in bottom of baking dish. Sprinkle breadcrumbs mixture over eggplant retaining just a little for the top of dish. Pour tomato sauce over eggplant and then top with mozzarella cheese slices. Sprinkle remaining breadcrumbs over cheese. Garnish with parsley flakes if desired. Bake 25 to 30 minutes.

Serves 4 – 160 calories per serving.

Stir Fry

Use an electric wok or a stir fry pan on the stove.

Shrimp or chicken

Broccoli

Cauliflower

Onion

Cabbage

Brussels sprouts

Carrots

Squash

Chop the vegetables in the amount you need for your family. Add 2 tbsp of olive oil to your pan. Put the meat in first and cook until nearly done. Add the vegetables. Stir constantly to prevent sticking. Prick the vegetables occasionally to test for doneness. Allow them to get crisp. Serve.

Vegetable Soup

1-28 oz can of tomatoes

1-15 oz can beef broth (not fat)

1 small pack frozen peas

1 small pack frozen corn

1 lb chopped carrots

1 bunch of celery

1 pack Lipton soup mix (Recipe secretes blue box)

1 Medium chopped onion

2 medium chopped potatoes

Water as needed

Add water to a boiler. Put the potatoes in boiler and cook until tender. Add vegetables. Season with a dash of salt, pepper and curry. Add beef broth. Reduce heat to simmer until vegetables are tender. Serve.

Left-over can be frozen and thawed as needed.

Chapter 5

Staying On Your Diet

Proven way to help you stay on your diet

Don't think about food; make an effort to avoid it. When a food commercial comes on television avoid watching it. Think about being thin and healthy.

Don't skip meals, you will only get hungry and eat too much.

Stay busy; work around the house, yard or other projects.

Plan your meals ahead of time; don't get caught short and hungry.

Keep fattening foods out of the house.

Always leave something on your plate.

Put your fork down between bites, while you chew slowly.

Beyond Weight Loss

If you are forced into a food encounter eat a small amount.

Do not combine eating with other activities such as watching TV.

Diet one day at a time, you can't eat for tomorrow until it gets here

Start some sort of exercise program and do it regularly.

Keep a record of what you eat, where you are, who you are with and what the occasion is.

Don't broadcast to the world that you are on a diet. Wait until you have had some measure of success. Some people are jealous of others trying to benefit and better themselves.

Don't let cheating blow your whole diet. Realize that you made a mistake and try to do better.

If you get to a point where you are not losing weight, it may be what is called a set point. When you reach at set point, the only thing to get you started again is aerobic exercise. That is exercise that you keep moving for a period of time. (Usually 15 minutes a day is sufficient.)

Imagine yourself thin.

Chapter 6

Exercise

You don't have to become a weight lifter or a try to build a Tarzan type body to lose weight. I developed a saying some years ago that went like this: "Mile by mile it's hard to smile, yard by yard may still be hard, but inch by inch it's a cinch."

An exercise program can be developed wherever you are and whatever you are doing. Simply walking is an excellent form of exercise.

Weight loss is all about burning more calories than you eat, but what's the best way to do that? Knowing the basics of how to lose weight, how to exercise for weight loss and how to motivate yourself are essential for creating a program that works for you. These resources will give you the tools you need to lose weight. Whether you're a beginner or you've been through the weight loss process before, you'll find everything you need to know about weight loss.

Too often we take drastic measures to see results -- diets, pills or those weird fitness gadgets on infomercials that promise instant success. Maybe you lose weight but what happens when you go off that diet or stop that crazy workout program? You gain it all back and more. The real secret to weight loss is to make small, lasting changes. The key is to forget about instant results and settle in for the long run.

If you've ever tried to lose weight, you know it can be a difficult process. But, there are ways to make it easier. Understanding exactly what you need to do to lose weight is your first step and these resources will help you learn about the basic steps to lose weight, how to set realistic goals and simple tips for making healthy lifestyle changes.

Remember the old saying, "If you always do what you have always done, you will always be what you have always been." You have to decide to do something different than you are now doing if you expect to lose weight.

General exercise may do for some while others may need to target certain areas of your body. If you have extra weight in your mid-section, butt or thighs you will need to work on those areas.

My suggestion is to start out walking. Read the next chapter on the psychology of weight loss and set a goal. Increase your distance as time goes by. Many health sources recommend walking 10,000 steps a day. I doubt that most people walk more than 3,000, which is way short of the goal. Get a pedometer, a devise that clips on your clothing, and see how many steps you are walking each day. I think you'll be surprised.

After a period of walking you may want to join a gym or club. They have experienced personnel to help you with any problems.

By all means, start slow and work up, and talk to your doctor.

Chapter 7

Psychological

Getting your attitude right may be more important than the food you eat or the exercise you get. Actually with the right attitude the other two will fall into place.

Let me explain what I mean. I teach using hypnosis for weight control. I have been a practicing hypnotist since 1976. I was meeting with a group of about 15 ladies. After a short lecture I would hypnotize the entire group at the same time. All the ladies were doing great; reporting weight loss every week, except one lady. She was beginning to get discouraged because the others were doing great and she had not lost any weight.

After two or three weeks I asked her to stay after the others left. I explained to her that there must be some psychological reason that she is not getting results like the others. I put her in a light trance and told her that she was walking down a hallway. On each side of the hallway there were many doors and behind one of these doors was the reason she was not responding. Slowly by my suggestions she would mentally open a door and see what was inside. After a few doors she said, I see it." I asked, "What do you see?" She exclaimed, "I see why I do not lose weight."

After awakening her I asked her to tell me what she saw. She said, "My husband is very jealous of me and I if I lose weight I would be attracted to other men and he would leave me. In order to keep my husband I have to stay fat."

I told her that there was nothing left that I could do. That is a personal problem and she would have to handle it herself.

There are many people who do not lose weight because of psychological problems. If you think you fit into this category you need to do some soul searching and find the answer, even if it means consulting a hypnotist. Later I will offer you some suggestion that might help you.

I had an interesting case when hypnotizing for weight control. This lady was a one-on-one case. We talked about her weight and what she was eating. She told me that she eats too much chocolate cake. I explained that the calories in the chocolate cake was enough to cause her to gain weight. When I finished I suggested that we enter a period of hypnosis. She said, "I don't need it. You told me what to do and I will do it." She never had a further problem with eating chocolate cake and she kept her weight under control.

In one of my earlier classes there was a young lady present. I only taught one class and never had further contact with most of them. I heard from the lady about a year later and she had lost 58 pounds.

No matter what you are trying to accomplish attitude is number one. Your attitude is what you think and how you feel. Attitudes can be changed instantly.

The Human Mind:

Let's take a look at how the human mind works. Like a computer that stores knowledge to provide answers, the mind consists of a brain and a nervous system to give the answers.

When information is fed into a mechanical computer, something comes out. Feed in a problem and receive an answer. The same thing is true of the brain. Everything that comes into our minds through the five senses ... everything that we see, hear, smell, taste and touch becomes a part of our subconscious mind ... our memory bank. When a problem is fed into our brain, the memory bank goes to work and returns the answer to us, through our nervous system.

The answer comes out in our characteristics: our personalities, the way we live and act, the clothes we wear, the house we live in the car we live. These are all a result of what has been fed into our individual – personal computer. There is no exception to this rule. Everything that goes in through the five senses determines our characteristics. It determines our personality.

If the answers coming out of our brain are less that our accomplishing potential, then we need to be very careful what we feed into it. We have to reprogram our computer. We need to grasp our automatic machine, the human mind, and do something about it.

Another way the human mind can be explained: There are two parts to it. First, there is the conscious. This is only a very small part of the brain. The purpose of the conscious mind is to censure, question and reject any and all information that goes into it. The conscious mind assimilates everything that we come in contact with and each thought we have. Whatever comes into our mind is questioned by the conscious mind. It rejects when it possible can.

The larger part of the brain is the subconscious. In some cases it is called the unconscious mind because it accepts everything as fact. It denies nothing. It does know a grey area, only black and white.

First of all, as we mentioned earlier, the conscious mind censors, rejects, questions all information that goes into it. When this process is complete, the thoughts are forwarded to the subconscious mind or the memory bank. They stay as long as we live. The significant information penetrates the subconscious mind and takes whatever steps are necessary to transform the thought into its physical equivalent.

If the thought is insignificant it places it into the memory bank and it is practically forgotten. Occasionally we may remember that particular thought, but seldom happens. Therefore, all conscious thought is censored before being placed into the subconscious mind.

There are times when we can bypass the conscious mind. One of these is through a state of deep relaxation, such as immediately before falling asleep at night. Or, we can place ourselves in this state by self-hypnosis. At these times, we can feed thoughts directly into our subconscious mind.

Throughout the following pages, you will learn ways to feed thoughts into your subconscious mind. When we program the subconscious mind, this is subliminal cybernetics in action.

The degree to which the suggestion is accepted depends on the degree to which the subconscious mind is receptive. And by this we mean: We must clear our minds of negative thoughts.

This book will teach you to do that very thing. You are going to learn how to rid yourself of the negative thoughts as soon as the doubt begins.

There are simple steps to remove these thoughts. When we free our minds of all negative; thoughts, doubts and fears, our minds become receptive to new and better ideas as fact and our minds will begin to take steps to make those things come true.

The mind obeys every suggestion that is verbalized! Remember this because this is important. Every suggestion that is said orally or verbalized, seen or visualized, felt or emotionalized is accepted by the subconscious mind.

When we verbalize a suggestion, the subconscious mind is more apt to pick it up and act on that suggestion. For example, we can think, "I ought to do a certain thing tomorrow." All we actually do is to think of this thing. On the other hand, we say to ourselves, "I am going to do a certain thing tomorrow." We repeat that thing to ourselves a few times and chances are, we are going to get out and do that thing we are talking about.

When we visualize ourselves doing that thing, then we are more likely to do it. When we emotionalize, in fact we put a great deal of emotion into our verbal suggestion, such as, "I've got faith in what I am going to do; "I've got faith in this thing that needs to be done, so tomorrow, I am going out and I am going to accomplish it." This is when we get emotional with ourselves.

When we combine these three, chances are that that deed will be accomplished. Sometimes we don't accomplish something because we simply don't have the courage to put it into words. We don't have enough gumption to state, firmly, "This is what I am going to do and nothing can stop me."

We can sit in our easy chair at home, close our eyes and actually see ourselves doing whatever we wanted to do, then combine it with a great deal of emotion and the chances are excellent that that deed will become a reality.

This is called packing ideas into the subconscious mind so strongly that it will take over and make that thing come true, whatever it happens to be.

For example, we may say to ourselves, "I have a headache." First of all the conscious mind picks it up and answers, "Ah, you don't have time for a headache. Forget it. You don't need a headache. You have too many things to do."

Soon after that you may say, "Oh, my head hurts so bad." Well the idea begins to seep through the conscious mind into the subconscious mind. We keep verbalizing, visualizing and emotionalizing until the subconscious take over … it make that thing come true … you have a splitting headache.

When you said, "I think I've got a headache," then you stated "I've got a headache." The subconscious mind picked that up and said, "He wants a headache, so let's give him one." And it happens.

Over-weight people think fat thoughts. To get your weight to where you want it to be you need to re-program your thinking. For instance: Put an empty picture frame in your bedroom where you can see it most often. Every time you see the frame see yourself as the size you want to be. See yourself dressed in the clothes you desire to wear. See yourself with a smile on your beautiful face. It works.

There are some other mental exercises you can do to get you

weight under control. Sit in a comfortable chair. Close your eyes and relax. Mentally think "I am very relaxed. My muscles are like a handful of rubber bands on a desk; loose, limp and relaxed." When you feel totally relaxed then say to yourself, "Every day in every way I am the size I want to be." As you think this picture yourself the size you want to be. Imagine that you are standing on a scale. The needle is pointing to the weight you intend to be. See yourself doing things that you have wanted to do. See yourself eating the proper foods. See yourself exercising with ease. See yourself as being happy.

Find time to go through this exercise daily if possible. It only takes as few minutes and easy to do.

What is Success?

Success in weight control is the journey to get to your desire weight, not after you get there. Think of success as a journey not a destination.

If success was measured by physical accomplishments, the person driving a Cadillac would be more successful than the driver of a Ford. And the driver of a Mercedes would be more successful than the one driving a Cadillac. The family who dines at the country club would be more successful than one who chooses to eat hamburgers or visit the Colonel for a chicken dinner.

When big goals are broken down into smaller goals — a day — an hour, and accomplished in small bits — that's success. The smaller accomplishments will lead to bigger accomplishments and finally, your ultimate dream.

Desire:

Success requires a strong desire. Two rival football teams were playing, the most important game of the season. One team was losing their best players to injures. In the 4th, quarter, the coach was about to give up, his best runner pulled a muscle in his leg. The crowd started shouting, "Bring in Leroy." The coach responded, "Leroy is not a football player, his on the track team." The crowd continued, "Who cares if he's not a football player, he can run." The game was getting down to the last few minutes. The coach decided to bring Leroy in.

A player attempted to give Leroy the ball. He refused to take it. The crowd was shouting, "Give the ball to Leroy, give the ball to Leroy." The coach had all he could stand. He took the ball over to the stand and throw the ball toward the fans and shouted, "Leroy don't want the ball."

Motivation:

We don't do anything until something motivates us to action. Success requires motivation. Why do you want to lose weight?

There are three types of motivation. The first is incentive. Incentive motivation requires an appetite. If you just finished a big meal and someone invites you to eat lunch with them, you would probably turn it down. You're not hungry. You don't have an appetite. You are not motivated to eat again.

Incentive motivation is like tying a carrot in front of a donkey. If he's hungry, he will pull the cart.

The next type of motivation is fear. Fear motivation is punishment for not doing something. When the boss says, "Get the job done, or else."

Fear motivation is like whipping the donkey to make him run and pull the cart. Fear motivation destroys initiative. This is trying to lose weight because your husband ordered you to do so, or threatened you if you didn't.

The third type of motivation is attitude. This is when you convince the donkey that he is a race horse. He will pull the cart because he wants to do it.

You have to want to lose weight because it will make you healthier and happier.

The company we mentioned earlier, ViSalus uses two of the above methods of motivation; incentive and attitude. They offer a 90 day challenge. The challenge is based on six points.

1 – 90 day money back results guarantee. You have nothing to lose but weight.

2 – During 2012 they gave over $47 million in free products, prizes and vacations.

3 – Project 10; every week in 2013 they are awarding a total of $10,000 to 10 people who lose 10 lbs.

4 – Monthly challenge finalist; Finalist will receive a professional photo shoot and free Vi-Gear.

5 – Ultimate transformation vacation; your before and after party, now with upgrade experiences and a $5,000 Beverly Hills Wardrobe Shopping Spree.

6 – Challenge trainer; every resource you need to succeed on your challenge, including challenge.com and other enhanced tools, apps and expert tips.

From the Challenge Magazine, volume 2 – issue 1 – 2013.

Reminder call Steve Holt 864-706-1428, ask him about the challenge.

Setting Goals:

A goal is defined as something you want; but it's more. Decide what you want, set a date for its attainment and map out a plan for the achievement and you have a goal.

The three parts of a goal as described above are absolutely necessary. Look at them one at a time. Know what you want. If you don't know what you want, how can you expect to get it? You might get it and didn't know you had it, if you didn't know you wanted it. Usually if you ask for nothing that's exactly what you will get.

Decide how much weight you want to lose. Goals must be realistic, measureable and reachable. Some people only want to lose five to ten pounds, while others want to lose 100 or more pounds. Only you can make this decision.

Formulate your goal into a paragraph. For instance: By _____ I will lose _____ pounds. I will do this by _____ (name the process you intend to use.) It is not a real goal until you have taken this step.

Create a Master Mind Group:

Have a few friends that you can confide in and will give you encouragement. Discuss your accomplishments and desire. Meet with them as often as possible. Never allow negative issues to be discussed.

Have Faith and Confidence:

Confidence is that ingredient that carries you through the rough spots. It gives you stamina, to keep going when weakness is about to overtake you. It gives you vision when the future looks foggy and dim. It gives you the courage to keep fighting when it looks like the fight is already lost.

Confidence can be gained at least two ways:

(1) From successful experiences. When doing a job well you have the confidence to try again. The first experience may be small and insignificant, but as you repeat the same experience, your confidence increases.

The baseball player gains confidence with each home run. The boxer gains confidence by winning one round at a time. The salesperson gains confidence by making one sale at a time. The young homemaker gains confidence when she bakes a cake and her family or friends tell how good it is.

When helping a person to build their confidence, never criticize anything they do. Criticism destroys initiative. Praise their good points and allow them to discover their own weaknesses. This, of course, does not eliminate the need for instruction.

(2) Confidence may be gain by visual imagery. It has been discovered that the mind cannot distinguish between an imaginary experience and an actual experience. This accounts for the tremendous number of mentally ill people. You can visualize a thing to be true and the mind will accept it as an actual event.

Faith is a state of mind which may be induced by repeated suggestion. You can build your faith by using positive affirmations. An affirmation is something that you affirm or declare to be so. An example might be, when you get up in the morning, you say, "Boy do I feel good." While repeating this statement, visualize the result and you have the visual assent. Now, combine these two with the emotion of faith. Anything you can visualize, verbalize and emotionalize long enough must inevitably happen.

Combat Fears and Doubts:

Fear is a state of mind, the complete opposite of faith. Fears and doubts are the most deadly weapons in destroying 100 or more pounds. Only you can make this decision.

Formulate your goal into a paragraph. For instance: By _____ I will lose _____ pounds. I will do this by _____ (name the process you intend to use.) It is not a real goal until you have taken this step.

Create a Master Mind Group:

Have a few friends that you can confide in and will give you encouragement. Discuss your accomplishments and desire. Meet with them as often as possible. Never allow negative issues to be discussed.

Have Faith and Confidence:

Confidence is that ingredient that carries you through the rough spots. It gives you stamina, to keep going when weakness is about to overtake you. It gives you vision when the future looks foggy and dim. It gives you the courage to keep fighting when it looks like the fight is already lost.

Confidence can be gained at least two ways:

(1) From successful experiences. When doing a job well you have the confidence to try again. The first experience may be small and insignificant, but as you repeat the same experience, your confidence increases.

The baseball player gains confidence with each home run. The boxer gains confidence by winning one round at a time. The salesperson gains confidence by making one sale at a time. The young homemaker gains confidence when she bakes a cake and her family or friends tell how good it is.

When helping a person to build their confidence, never criticize anything they do. Criticism destroys initiative. Praise their good points and allow them to discover their own weaknesses. This, of course, does not eliminate the need for instruction.

(2) Confidence may be gain by visual imagery. It has been discovered that the mind cannot distinguish between an imaginary experience and an actual experience. This accounts for the tremendous number of mentally ill people. You can visualize a thing to be true and the mind will accept it as an actual event.

Faith is a state of mind which may be induced by repeated suggestion. You can build your faith by using positive affirmations. An affirmation is something that you affirm or declare to be so. An example might be, when you get up in the morning, you say, "Boy do I feel good." While repeating this statement, visualize the result and you have the visual assent. Now, combine these two with the emotion of faith. Anything you can visualize, verbalize and emotionalize long enough must inevitably happen.

Combat Fears and Doubts:

Fear is a state of mind, the complete opposite of faith. Fears and doubts are the most deadly weapons in destroying the mind of man. They destroy desire, initiative and hope for better things in the future.

Fear and doubt, being states of mind, can be fought by inducing repeated suggestions. Should you find yourself thinking, "I'm afraid I can't do that," your subconscious mind will accept the request as, "I don't want to do it," and will help to bring it into reality.

Create an Obsession for your Goal:

An obsession, being described as a burning desire, is the success ingredient that burns the path to your goal.

There are seven steps necessary in becoming obsessed enough to do anything you desire or in becoming the person you wish to be.

(1) Write out your major, definite goal. State when you intend to do to get it.

(2) Write a plan for the attainment of your goal. When a pilot departs from one airport he makes a flight chart. He knows where he is going, when he expects to get there and the route he will follow. This is much the same as a plan for attaining a personal goal.

(3) Read your statement aloud several times a day. You should repeat your main goal at least 50 times a day. This may be done while driving to work or at any time you have a few minutes to concentrate.

(4) Record your goals on a cassette player and listen to them twice daily, morning and evening.

(5) Gather pictures and clippings to remind you of your goal. Place them in conspicuous places such as: the bathroom mirror, the sun visor of your car, or wherever you will see them most often.

(6) Spend some time each day visualizing your goals. See

the final results. Picture all the details. See yourself as if you had already accomplished the thing you want.

(7) Expect results. The power of expectation is greater than science or psychological research has discovered. Often it is the reason things get done, but the lack of understanding has allowed other phases of research to get the glory.

My favorite expression is: "When you pray for rain, take an umbrella."

Specialize in Knowledge Pertinent to your goal:

In the age of specialization, general knowledge is not sufficient to reach outstanding accomplishments.

Your special knowledge should be learning more about food and ways of exercising. Learn different recipes that keep the intake according to your limits.

Stick-Ability and Persistence:

The ability to keep going in the threat of possible failure is what separates the strong from the weak. One is not a failure until he has accepted it in his own mind. History is filled with heroes who refused to give up.

Should you make a mistake and eat too much, don't let that derail your plans. The next day do a better job and forget about the past.

There is one major difference in success and failure. The successful ones keep going when the failures give up too soon.

You can be the person you want to be.

Chapter 8

Learn Self-Hypnosis

Hypnosis is can be very valuable in your weight control program. It can be done with the aid of someone to guide you or you can learn to do it yourself.

Recently, I had a bone biopsy done. The doctor warned me that the procedure was painful. He explained that he would use a very long needle and force it into a bone in my back. While he was out of the room, I quickly hypnotized myself and suggested that during the procedure I would remain free of pain. As he forced the needle into my spine, he kept apologizing for the pain. At times he stopped to make sure I was ok. When he finished he was baffled that I took the pain so easily. I explained that I used hypnosis. He was in disbelief.

The followings suggestions will help to guide you through a hypnotic trance.

Get Comfortable - Look forward, breathe slowly and easily, relax. Don't cross your legs or arms.

Repeat to yourself (mentally), I am totally relaxed. Never have I been so relaxed. Feel your body beginning to get heavy. Reach a total state of relaxation. Give yourself ample time to get relaxed.

State your goal - Tell yourself your purpose in going into self hypnosis. "I am going into a trance for the purpose of _____ . (*Filling in the blank with what you want to achieve.*) During this self-hypnosis session my unconscious mind will make the adjustments so that _____ (*Filling in the blank with what you want to achieve*) occurs naturally and easily.

How To Feel Afterward - Tell yourself how you want to feel when you complete the process and how long you wish to be in a trance, "In twenty minutes, I'm going to feel _____".

Keep all suggestions positive. For instance: Don't say, "I am not going to eat fattening foods." Rather say, "I am eating foods that are healthy for my body. Never use negatives.

Take your time. Make suggestions slowly, with rhythm.

If you don't get all the way through, relax. In fact, it's a sign that you've gone deep enough if you lose track of where you are in the process. Just let your mind wander where it will and trust that your unconscious is carrying out the suggestions you gave it.

Allow yourself to come out of trance whenever it feels appropriate. You'll often find that you come out very near the time you suggested.

This will take practice. Be patience. You will become better and more efficient each time you go under.

You may prefer to use a cassette tape and record your suggestions. Choose a location where you will not be disturbed. Have a script ready and read the suggestions. Talk slowly and with rhythm. In the beginning, this is something you will have to practice a lot. Use a personal application and make it present. I am, not I will.

When you are ready to use the tape, turn the tape player on and just relax. Listen to the words being said. Let the tape work for you.

Make a different tape for each situation. For instance: don't include stop smoking and weight loss on the same tape.

You make choose to use the following script:

I am in a complete state of relaxation. My body is relaxing more and more. Never have I been so relaxed, in all my lifetime, as I am right now. My body is feeling heaver and heaver. All the muscles in my body are relaxed. More and more relaxed. Completely and totally relaxed. I am imagining that I am riding down and escalator (like the ones in a department store.) As I go down I will count from 20 to one. When I reach one, I will be at the bottom. At the bottom I will be in a complete state of hypnotic sleep. 20 down, down, down. 19 down, down, down. 18 down, down, down. 17 down, down, down. 16 down, down, down. 15 down, down, down. 14 down, down, down. 13 down, down, down. 12 down, down, down. 11 down, down, down. 10 down, down, down. 9 down, down, down. 10 down, down, down. 9 down, down, down. 8 down, down, down. 7 down, down, down. 6 down, down, down. 5 down, down, down. 4 down, down, down. 3 down, down, down. 2 down, down, down. 1 down, down, down. I am completely and totally relaxed. I am now in a very relaxed state and in hypnotic sleep. I am going to make myself some suggestions. From this day forward...

Here insert your own suggestions. Assuming you want to

gain confidence, try this.

I am free of negative thoughts. I am free of all fears. I can do anything I choose. My confidence is growing day by day. My nerves are like a piece of steel. I am free of doubts. My future is bright. My hopes are positive. My dreams are becoming very clear. I expect good things to happen to me. I feel great. I feel wonderful. Never have I felt so good in all my lifetime, as I do right now.

You have a choice to awaken yourself or go into natural sleep. Should you choose to play the tape when you go to bed, you will want to let yourself go into natural sleep. Your suggestions would be like this:

I am now going to sleep for the night. As I go into natural sleep, my body is relaxing more, and more.

Let the tape shut itself off and relax.

Chapter 8

Foods That Heal

The chances are most likely that if you have been overweight for a period of time you are suffering from one or more disease. This chapter is a quick reference to most common diseases and food that have been known to heal the disease. Eating right, getting exercise and rest will help you to live a longer and a more productive life. Individuals can help to live healthier, however consult your doctor for specific problems.

We suggest that you keep this book handy to be used as an aid in knowing which foods to buy.

90

Diseases and the Foods
To Eat to Heal Them

ARTHRITIS AND INFLAMMATION: Fish with omega 3; tuna, salmon, sardine & mackerel.

ACNE: Fresh fruits and vegetables, Vitamins A, B, C and zinc. Whole grains and cereals lean meat, poultry, and fish.

AIDS/HIV INFECTIONS: Meat, liver, eggs, milk, high protein foods, pasta and other starchy foods, cooked vegetables, and pasteurized juices and canned fruits.

ALZHEIMER'S DISEASE: Eggs, liver, soy products, whole-grains and wheat germ.

ANEMIA: Organ meats, beef, poultry, egg yolks, B-12, Fried beans, soy products, dates, raisins, dried apricots, blackstrap molasses, breads, cereal, citrus fruits, and green leafy vegetables.

APPETITE LOSS: Fresh fruits and vegetables lean meats, seafood, poultry, nuts and whole-grains.

ARTHRITIS: Salmon, sardines, mackerel, tuna, and fresh high fiber foods.

ASTHMA: Chicken soup, broth and omega 3.

ARTERIOSCLEROSIS: Fresh fruits and vegetables, wheat germ, lean poultry, seafood, vitamin E, salmon, sardines and omega 3.

BAD BREATH: Water, fruit juices and sour foods.

BLEEDING PROBLEMS: Spinach, potatoes, cabbage, whole

grains, organ meats, lean meats, poultry, seafood, Vitamin B-12, Citrus and other fresh fruits and vegetables.

BLOOD PRESSURE: Celery and other fresh vegetables, fresh and dried fruits, oats cereals and legumes.

BULIMIA: Fresh fruits and vegetables, high fiber foods, bananas, dried fruits and grains.

BURNS: Lean meats, poultry, shellfish, eggs, legumes, water, broth, juices, fresh fruits and vegetables.

CANCER: Citrus fruits, dark green and yellow vegetables, cauliflower, whole grain breads and high fiber foods.

CHRONIC FATIGUE SYNDROME: Pasta, rice, whole grain cereal and breads, lean meat, fish, poultry, fresh fruits and vegetables and salty foods if blood pressure is low.

CIRCULATION DISORDERS: Salmon, sardines, oily fish, omega 3, citrus and other fresh fruits and vegetables, seeds, nuts, seafood, wheat germ and vitamin E.

CIRRHOSIS: Grains and legumes instead of meats for protein, carbohydrates, cereals, breads, Potatoes, B-complex vitamins and fresh fruits and vegetables.

COLDS & FLU: Fresh fruits and vegetables, wheat germ, dried peas, and beans, seafood, meat, zinc, garlic, hot peppers and fluids.

COLITIS: Poached fruits, steamed vegetables, eggs, fish, poultry, lean meats, Protein and iron.

CONSTIPATION: Fresh fruits and vegetables, grains and fluids (at least 8 glasses per day.)

CRAVINGS: Low-fat starchy foods, and high fiber foods.

CROHN'S DISEASE: Lean meats, fish and poultry.

CYSTIC FIBROSIS: Fish, poultry, eggs, meat, starchy foods, fat, and salt fluids.

DEHYDRATION: Water, juices, milk, fresh fruits and vegetables.

DENTAL DISORDERS: Low-fat milk, yogurt, cheese, fresh fruits and vegetables, and vitamins A & C.

DEPRESSION: Meat, eggs, dairy products, and fish.

DIABETES: Eat regular meals, starches, proteins and fat with each meal, fruits, and high fiber foods.

DIARRHEA: Water, mineral water, herbal tea, ginger ale, apple juice, broth, low sugar sports beverages, skinless baked potato, boiled and poached eggs.

DIGESTIVE DISORDERS: Fresh fruits and vegetables, whole grain products, and fluids (at least 8 glasses per day).

DIVERTICULITIS: Seedless fresh fruits and vegetables, whole grain cereals and bread.

DRY MOUTH: Fluids such as water, juice and tea, Fruits and sherbet puddings.

EAR DISORDERS: Plenty of fresh fruits and vegetables.

ECZEMA: Legumes, fresh fruits and vegetables.

EYE DISORDERS: Carrots, sweet potatoes, dark green vegetables, citrus fruits, melons, tomatoes, vitamin C, whole grains, seeds, nuts, avocados, potatoes, bananas, fish, poultry, lean meats, Vitamin B, legumes, dried fruit, seafood, lean meats and eggs.

FOOD POISONING: Diluted sweetened drinks, bananas, rice, cooked apples and dried toast.

FRACTURES: Low-fat milk, dairy products, sardines with bones, fortified milk, eggs, liver and oily fish.

GALLSTONES: Small meals at regular times and breakfast daily.

GASTRITIS: Regular balanced meals with starchy foods, fresh fruits and vegetables and low-fat protein.

GOUT: Plenty of fluids, fresh fruits and vegetables, cereals, pasta and rice.

HAIR & SCALP PROBLEMS: Low-fat dairy products, dark green vegetables, fruits, whole grain products, bananas, prunes, watermelon, nuts, legumes, lean meats, poultry and fish.

HAY FEVER: Salmon, Mackerel, tuna and omega 3.

HEART DISEASE: Fresh fruits and vegetables, foods with vitamin C, poultry, seafood, wheat germ, fortified cereals, vitamin E, Apples, oat bran and fiber foods.

HERPES: Lamb, chicken, fish, beans, fruits and vegetables.

HIATAL HERNIA: High fiber foods such as whole grain cereals and breads, fresh fruits, salads, and raw or lightly cooked vegetables.

HIVES: Fortified cereals and breads, fish, poultry, and other niacin -rich foods.

HYPERACTIVITY: A variety of foods to provide a nutritional complete diet.

HYPOGLYCEMIA: Small meals that provide a balance of protein, carbohydrates and fats.

IMPOTENCE: Foods rich in zinc, such as yogurt, fortified cereals, wheat germ, vegetables, shellfish and poultry.

INDIGESTION AND HEARTBURN: Small meals at regular intervals.

INFERTILITY: Fish, shellfish, lean meat, legumes, fortified bread, vitamins B, iron, zinc, fresh fruits and vegetables, dairy products, wheat germ, seeds, eggs, poultry, sea food and vitamin E.

INTOLERANCE TO MILK: Lactose-reduced milk lactase enzyme tablets, cheese, and yogurt.

IRRITABLE BOWEL SYNDROME: Nonalcoholic, caffeine-free fluids, smaller meals, high fiber foods (if constipation is a problem) and binding foods (if diarrhea is a problem).

JUNDICE: Lean meats, poultry, fish, low-fat dairy products, eggs, and low-fat foods high in protein.

KIDNEY DISEASE: Liquids to replace lost fluids and maintain fluid balance.

LIVER DISEASE: Fish, dark green vegetables, beans, omega 3, fresh fruits and vegetables and legumes.

LUNG DISORDERS: Non-alcoholic fluids, fresh fruits and vegetables, vitamin E, nuts, seeds, eggs, vitamin E, lean meats, oysters, yogurt, whole grain products and zinc.

LUPUS: Grapefruit, broccoli, cabbage, kale, whole grain products, Vitamin E, zinc, selenium and plant seed oils.

MENOPAUSE: Foods high in calcium and vitamin D, low-fat dairy products, dark leafy vegetables, legumes, fiber products and fresh fruits and vegetables.

MIGRAINES AND OTHER HEADACHES: Cut down on coffee, tea, and other beverages containing caffeine. Avoid alcohol and red wine.

MONONUCLEOUSIS: Fruit and vegetable juices, milk shakes, vitamin D, soups and soft foods to soothe a sore throat.

MOOD DISORDERS: A variety of complex carbohydrates, seafood, dark leafy vegetables, whole grain breads and cereals, and pasta.

MULTIPLE SCLEROSIS: High fiber foods, cranberry juice and pureed foods.

MUSCLE CRAMPS: Low-fat dairy products, bananas, citrus fruits, dried fruits, tomato juice, deep yellow vegetables, walnuts, pecans, sunflower seeds, rice, legumes, pasta, whole-grain breads and cereals, water and B-complex vitamins.

NAIL PROBLEMS: Lean meat, poultry, fish, Protein, citrus fruits, dark green leafy vegetables whole grain products, legumes, fruits juices and B-vitamins.

NEURALGIA: Lean meats, poultry, eggs, low-fat dairy products, fortified breads and cereals, spinach, potatoes, poultry, nuts, melons, seafood, nuts, seeds, wheat germ and whole grain foods.

OBESITY: Plenty liquids, complex carbohydrates, potatoes, rice, legumes, whole grain foods, fresh fruits and vegetables, fiber, multiple-vitamins, fish, skinless poultry and low-fat dairy products.

ORAL THRUSH: Lean meats, fish, fortified breads and cereals, dried fruits, and raw garlic.

OSTEOPOROSIS: Low-fat milk, yogurt, canned fish with bones, oily fish, fortified dairy products and legumes.

PALPITATIONS: Eat foods that are high in potassium and magnesium.

PARKINSON'S DISEASE: Fresh fruits and vegetables, whole grain products, fluids and soft or pureed foods.

PREGNANCY: Lean meats, poultry, fish, dried beans, lentils, eggs, milk, dairy products, canned sardines and salmon, both with bones, citrus fruits, dark green leafy vegetables. Legumes, whole grains and fortified cereals.

PROSTATE PROBLEMS: Tomatoes, red grapefruits, watermelons, vegetable oils, margarine, wheat germ, whole grain products, nuts, seeds, fresh fruits and vegetables, fish shellfish, lean meats, yogurt, legumes, zinc and fluids.

SCHIZOPHRENIA: A combination of animal protein and starchy foods.

SEX DRIVE: Legumes, fortified grains and cereals, poultry, wheat germ, dark green leafy vegetables, vitamin B, fresh fruits and vegetables, poultry, seafood, lean meats, fish, yogurt, grains and oysters.

SHINGLES: Olive and other vegetable oils, nuts, seeds, wheat germ and fresh fruits and vegetables.

SINUSITIS: Fresh fruits and vegetables, whole grain products, legumes, nuts, vitamin B, sunflower seeds, vegetable oils, avocados, vitamins E, garlic and onions.

SKIN PROBLEMS: Yellow fruits and vegetables, dark leafy vegetables, vitamins A & C, legumes, whole grains, fortified breads and cereals, eggs, seafood, poultry, grains, zinc, oily fish and omega 3.

SORE THROATS: Citrus and other fresh fruits and vegetables, oranges, seafood, lean meats, yogurt and fortified grains.

STROKE: Fresh fruits and vegetables, nuts, seeds, green leafy vegetables, wheat germ, fortified cereal, bananas, oily fish, omega 3, oat bran, legumes, onions and garlic.

THYROID DISORDERS: Seafood, dark green leafy vegetables, deep yellow or orange fruits and vegetables, fortified cereals, low-fat dairy products and vitamin- A.

TUBERCULOSIS: Lean meat, poultry eggs, fish, legumes, pasta, fresh fruits and vegetables, fatty fish, grains, spinach, potatoes, shellfish, fortified cereals and bread, and zinc.

ULCERS: Lean meat, poultry, fortified cereals and bread, seafood, dried fruits and citrus fruits.

UNDER WEIGHT: Large portions of high calorie foods and nutritious snacks between meals.

URINARY TRACT INFECTIONS: Nonalcoholic and caffeine-free drinks, cranberry juice, blueberries, citrus and other fresh fruits and vegetables, high calcium foods and low-fat dairy products.

VAGINITIS: Dairy products, eggs, green and yellow vegetables, orange fruits, fish, vitamins A & D, fortified grains and cereals, poultry, seafood, bananas, dark green leafy vegetables, nuts, seeds, shellfish, beans, legumes and zinc.

VERTIGO: Low-fat high fiber foods.

WORMS AND OTHER PARASITES: Lean meats, poultry, seafood, legumes, citrus and other fresh fruits and vegetables, animal products and vitamin B-12.

Annotation

Just a few more words of advice which may be the most important part of the book.

I am type-2 diabetic and have been for 12 years. Recently I discussed my medication with my family doctor. He have me a lecture about what I eat. He said it's not totally the sweets you eat it's the starches.

He went on to say, "Stop taking your medication for one month and don't eat any starches. No carbohydrates? That's a tall order.

He said, "Leave off bread of any kind, cereal, grits, pasta, candy, cakes, pies and dried beans." I said if I leave off bread and all the things you mentioned, what do I eat for breakfast since it's the most important meal of the day for diabetics? He said go back to what they said would kill us 30 years ago; bacon and eggs.

My thoughts were that's disgusting. Eggs with no bread and jelly.

I decided to used his advice. Now I eat eggs with no bread. I stopped eating sandwiches, snack cakes, etc.

When my wife eats a sandwich I eat basically the same except no bread. My diabetes is under control with no medication.

If you are trying to control your weight the same diet will work for you. You don't need a magic pill, or any of the popular weight loss products on the market. They work for some because of the hype from the company. When the hype is gone the weight will come back.

If you want to lose weight you have to change your life-style. As we said before, "If you do what you've always done, you will always be what you've always been."

List of foods high in Carbohydrates
(Carb Calories per Serving)

Baked potato, Russet, baked (1 small potato, 5 oz.)   120

Waffles, Aunt Jemima (1 piece) 52

Gatorade (1 cup) 60

Grapenuts (approx. 1 cup, Kraft) 88

Bread, whole wheat (1 slice) 52

Bread, white (1 slice) 56

Bagel, (white, frozen) 140

Stuffing (approx. 1 cup) 84

Graham wafers (approx. 1 cup) 72

Grapenuts (approx. 1 cup, Kraft) 44

Shredded wheat (1 oz. serving) 80

Total (1 oz. serving, General Mills) 88

Cream of Wheat (1 oz. serving, instant, Nabisco) 120

 Spaghetti, (plain, cooked, 3/4 cup) 176

Rice (brown, cooked, 3/4 cup) 152

Raisin bran (1 oz. serving, Kellogg's) 76

Oatmeal (1 cup) 104

Bran muffin (large) 96

 Green pea soup (1 cup) 124

Ice cream, regular (1/2 cup) 52
Blueberry muffin (1) 116
Raisins (1/4 cup) 180
Powerbar, chocolate 104
Apple 64
Orange 44
Banana 96
Grapes (1 cup) 72
Carrot (raw, 1 medium) 36
Sweet corn (1/2 cup 68
Bread, 100% whole grain (1 slice) 52
Dried apricots (1/4 cup) 82
Peas (1/2 cup) 28
Orange juice (3/4 cup, 6 oz.) 92
Fruit yogurt (reduced fat, 3/4 cup) 96
Tomato soup (1 cup) 68
Skim milk (1 cup) 52
Baked beans (1/2 cup) 60
Lentils (1/2 cup) 76
Kidney beans (1/2 cup) 100
Lima beans (1/2 cup, baby, frozen) 120
Garbanzo beans (1/2 cup) 120

Some reading this are probably saying, "I can't live without my bread or some other food." It may be a question, "Would you rather live without bread or die fat and disease?"

Being overweight limits your ability to do many things such as; enjoy the kids while they are young, doing your house work without the pain, and a thousand other activities. Over weight shortens your life span, medical bills cost more and causes pain and suffering needlessly.

I have to insert one more suggestion: Throw away your salt shaker. According to nutritionists, small amounts of salt on a daily basis is essential for the functioning of healthy cells. Sodium - better known as salt - maintains the correct balance of certain fluids which bathe the cells in our bodies - essential for nerve and muscle function.

However, research shows that too much salt can lead to increased blood pressure, osteoporosis - a bone-thinning disease, asthma, stomach cancer and weight gain. Salt also causes:

Hypertension

Osteoporosis

Kidney problems

 Asthma

Stomach cancer

Weight gain

So can you live without a lot of salt? If you want to live a long life you can.

List of Foods and the
Amount of Starch in Each

1 Rice, white, long-grain, parboiled, unenriched, cooked - Starch: 47g
2 Rice, white, long-grain, precooked or instant, enriched, pre-

pared - Starch: 45g

3 Snacks, potato chips, fat-free, made with olestra - Starch: 42g

4 Rice, white, steamed, Chinese restaurant - Starch: 42g

5 Potatoes, russet, flesh and skin, raw - Starch: 40g

6 Potato, flesh and skin, raw - Starch: 40g

7 Cornmeal, degermed, enriched, white or yellow - Starch: 40g

8 Potatoes, mashed, dehydrated, flakes without milk, dry - Starch: 40g

9 Potatoes, white, flesh and skin, raw - Starch: 39g

10 Rice, white, long-grain, precooked or instant, enriched, dry - Starch: 39g

11 Cereals ready-to-eat, wheat, shredded, plain, sugar and salt free [Kraft, POST Shredded Wheat] - Starch: 39g

12 Potatoes, white, flesh and skin, baked - Starch: 38g

13 Cereals ready-to-eat, KELLOGG, KELLOGG'S Corn Flakes - Starch: 38g

14 Snacks, pretzels, hard, plain, salted - Starch: 38g

15 Corn flour, whole-grain - Starch: 37g

16 Cereals ready-to-eat, KELLOGG, KELLOGG'S RICE KRISPIES - Starch: 37g

17 Potato, baked, flesh and skin, without salt - Starch: 37g

18 Wheat flour, white (industrial), 9% protein, bleached, enriched - Starch: 37g

19 Snacks, potato chips, made from dried potatoes, fat-free - Starch: 36g

20 Tortilla, includes plain and from mutton sandwich (Navajo) - Starch: 36g

21 Wheat flour, white (industrial), 10% protein, bleached, enriched - Starch: 35g

22 Wheat flour, white (industrial), 10% protein, unbleached, enriched - Starch: 35g

23 Tennis Bread, plain (Apache) - Starch: 35g

24 Corn, sweet, yellow, frozen, kernels cut off cob, unprepared - Starch: 34g

25 Bagels, plain, enriched, with calcium propionate (includes onion, poppy, sesame) - Starch: 34g

26 Cereals ready-to-eat, Ralston Corn Flakes - Starch: 34g

27 Macaroni, dry, enriched - Starch: 34g

28 Macaroni, dry, unenriched - Starch: 34g

29 Spaghetti, dry, enriched or unenriched - Starch: 34g

30 Spaghetti, cooked, enriched, with added salt - Starch: 33g

31 English muffins, plain, toasted, enriched, with calcium propionate (includes sourdough) - Starch: 33g

32 Macaroni, cooked, enriched or unenriched - Starch: 33g

33 Spaghetti, cooked, enriched, without added salt - Starch: 33g

34 Wheat flour, white (industrial), 15% protein, bleached, enriched - Starch: 33g

35 English muffins, plain, enriched, with ca prop (includes sourdough) - Starch: 33g

36 Cereals, oats, regular and quick and instant, unenriched, cooked with water (includes boiling and microwaving), with salt - Starch: 33g

37 Cereals, oats, regular and quick and instant, unenriched, cooked with water (includes boiling and microwaving), without salt [oatmeal, cooked] - Starch: 33g

38 Snacks, popcorn, unpopped kernels - Starch: 32g

39 Cornmeal, yellow (Navajo) - Starch: 32g

40 Corn, sweet, yellow, canned, whole kernel, drained solids - Starch: 32g

41 Crackers, saltines (includes oyster, soda, soup) - Starch: 32g

42 Crackers, saltines, low salt (includes oyster, soda, soup) - Starch: 32g

43 Cereals ready-to-eat, GENERAL MILLS, KIX - Starch: 32g

44 Cereals ready-to-eat, Ralston Enriched Bran flakes - Starch: 31g

45 Cereals, oats, regular and quick and instant, not fortified, dry [oatmeal, old-fashioned oats, rolled oats] - Starch: 31g

46 Bread, white, commercially prepared (includes soft bread crumbs) Starch: 31g

47 Cereals, oats, instant, fortified, plain, prepared with water (boiling water added or microwaved) [instant oatmeal] - Starch: 31g

48 Cereals ready-to-eat, GENERAL MILLS, CHEERIOS - Starch: 30g

49 Bread crumbs, dry, grated, plain - Starch: 30g

50 Potatoes, french fried, all types, salt added in processing, frozen, home-prepared, oven heated - Starch: 30g

51 Snacks, popcorn, microwave, 94% fat free - Starch: 30g

52 Soup, wonton, Chinese restaurant - Starch: 30g

53 Sweet potato, raw, unprepared - Starch: 29g

54 Rolls, hamburger or hotdog, plain - Starch: 29g

55 Snacks, RALSTON PURINA, CHEX MIX - Starch: 28g

56 Snacks, popcorn, air-popped - Starch: 28g

57 Pancakes, plain, frozen, ready-to-heat, microwave (includes buttermilk) - Starch: 28g

58 - Corn, yellow, whole kernel, frozen, microwaved - Starch: 28g

59 Soup, chicken noodle, dry, mix - Starch: 27g

60 Babyfood, cereal, oatmeal, dry - Starch: 27g

61 Waffle, buttermilk, frozen, ready-to-heat, microwaved - Starch: 27g

62 Cereals ready-to-eat, KRAFT, POST GRAPE-NUTS Cereal - Starch: 27g

63 English muffins, raisin-cinnamon (includes apple-cinnamon) - Starch: 26g

64 English muffins, raisin-cinnamon, toasted (includes apple-cinnamon) - Starch: 26g

65 Cereals ready-to-eat, KRAFT, POST, HONEY BUNCHES OF OATS, honey roasted - Starch: 26g

66 Taco shells, baked - Starch: 25g

67 Snacks, tortilla chips, plain, yellow corn - Starch: 24g

68 Potatoes, french fried, crinkle or regular cut, salt added in processing, frozen, oven-heated - Starch: 24g

69 Cereals ready-to-eat, KELLOGG, KELLOGG'S FROSTED FLAKES - Starch: 24g

70 Macaroni and Cheese, canned entrée - Starch: 24g

71 Potatoes, french fried, shoestring, salt added in processing, frozen, oven-heated - Starch: 23g

72 Corned beef and potatoes in tortilla (Apache) - Starch: 23g

73 BURGER KING, French Fries - Starch: 23g

74 Cereals ready-to-eat, KELLOGG, KELLOGG'S COCOA

KRISPIES - Starch: 23g

75 Potato puffs, frozen, unprepared - Starch: 23g

76 Beans, navy, mature seeds, cooked, boiled, with salt - Starch: 22g

78 Beans, navy, mature seeds, cooked, boiled, without salt - Starch: 22g

79 Salad dressing, french dressing, fat-free - Starch: 22g

80 Refried beans, canned, fat-free - Starch: 22g

81 Snacks, tortilla chips, ranch-flavor - Starch: 22g

82 WENDY'S, French Fries - Starch: 22g

83 Beans, kidney, red, mature seeds, canned - Starch: 22g

84 Snacks, FRITOLAY, SUNCHIPS, Multigrain Snack, original flavor - Starch: 22g

85 DOMINO'S 14" Cheese Pizza, Classic Hand-Tossed Crust - Starch: 22g

86 Beans, pinto, mature seeds, cooked, boiled, with salt - Starch: 21g

87 Beans, kidney, all types, mature seeds, canned - Starch: 21g

88 NABISCO, NABISCO RITZ Crackers - Starch: 21g

89 Egg rolls, vegetable, refrigerated, heated - Starch: 21g

90 Snacks, tortilla chips, nacho cheese - Starch: 21g

91 TACO BELL, Bean Burrito - Starch: 21g

92 Pie crust, refrigerated, regular, baked - Starch: 20g

93 Spaghetti, no meat, canned - Starch: 20g

94 Cereals ready-to-eat, KELLOGG, KELLOGG'S APPLE JACKS - Starch: 20g

95 Crackers, standard snack-type, regular - Starch: 20g

96 Cereals ready-to-eat, KELLOGG, KELLOGG'S FROOT LOOPS - Starch: 20g

97 KENTUCKY FRIED CHICKEN, Potato Wedges - Starch: 20g

98 KENTUCKY FRIED CHICKEN - Starch: 20g

99 Cereals ready-to-eat, KELLOGG, KELLOGG'S RAISIN BRAN - Starch: 19g

100 LITTLE CAESARS 14" Original Round Cheese Pizza, Regular Crust - Starch: 19g

101 Lasagna with meat & sauce, low-fat, frozen entrée - Starch:

19g

102 PAPA JOHN'S 14" Cheese Pizza, Original Crust - Starch: 18g

103 Crackers, cheese, sandwich-type with cheese filling - Starch: 18g

104 Soup, egg drop, Chinese restaurant - Starch: 18g

105 Salad dressing, thousand island dressing, fat-free - Starch: 18g

106 Beans, baked, canned, with pork and tomato sauce - Starch: 17g

107 Cereals ready-to-eat, KELLOGG, KELLOGG'S ALL-BRAN Original - Starch: 17g

108 Toaster pastries, fruit, toasted (include apple, blueberry, cherry, strawberry) - Starch: 17g

109 TACO BELL, Nachos - Starch: 17g

110 Crackers, standard snack-type, sandwich, with peanut butter filling - Starch: 17g

111 Cereals ready-to-eat, GENERAL MILLS, LUCKY CHARMS - Starch: 16g

112TACO BELL, BURRITO SUPREME with steak - Starch: 16g

113 Cereals ready-to-eat, GENERAL MILLS, CINNAMON TOAST CRUNCH - Starch: 16g

114 Fast foods, hamburger; single, regular patty; with condiments - Starch: 16g

115 WENDY'S, Jr. Hamburger, without cheese - Starch: 16g

116 Sweet potato, cooked, baked in skin, without salt - Starch: 16g

117 BURGER KING, Hamburger - Starch: 15g

118 Sweet potato, cooked, baked in skin, with salt - Starch: 15g

119 Fish, fish portions and sticks, frozen, preheated - Starch: 15g

120 WENDY'S, Homestyle Chicken Fillet Sandwich - Starch: 15g

121 WENDY'S, Ultimate Chicken Grill Sandwich - Starch: 15g

122 Fast Foods, crispy chicken filet sandwich, with lettuce, to-

mato and mayonnaise - Starch: 15g

123 Fast foods, miniature cinnamon rolls - Starch: 14g

124 BURGER KING, Original Chicken Sandwich - Starch: 14g

125 Beans, baked, canned, with pork and sweet sauce - Starch: 14g

126 WENDY'S, Jr. Hamburger, with cheese -Starch: 13g

127 Beef Pot Pie, frozen entree, prepared - Starch: 13g

128 Bananas, raw - Starch: 12g

129 Spaghetti, with meatballs, canned - Starch: 12g

130 Fast foods, english muffin, with cheese and sausage - Starch: 12g

131 Fast foods, biscuit, with egg, cheese, and bacon - Starch: 12g

Click to view menu

132 TACO BELL, Taco Salad - Starch: 11g

133 Cookies, chocolate chip, commercially prepared, regular, higher fat, enriched - Starch: 11g

134 Chicken breast tenders, cooked, conventional oven - Starch: 11g

135 Fast foods, hamburger; single, large patty; with condiments, vegetables and mayonnaise - Starch: 11g

136 Cucumber, with peel, raw - Starch: 11g

137 Cookies, chocolate sandwich, with creme filling, regular - Starch: 11g

138 Peas, green, frozen, unprepared - Starch: 11g

139 WENDY'S, CLASSIC SINGLE Hamburger, no cheese - Starch: 11g

140 Snacks, granola bars, soft, uncoated, chocolate chip - Starch: 11g

141 Fast Foods, biscuit, with egg and sausage - Starch: 10g

142 Formulated bar, POWER BAR, chocolate - Starch: 10g

143 Cake, snack cakes, creme-filled, sponge - Starch: 9g

144 Chili con carne with beans, canned entrée - Starch: 9g

145 Pie, pumpkin, commercially prepared - Starch: 9g

146 Pie, pecan, commercially prepared - Starch: 8g

147 Nuts, cashew nuts, oil roasted, with salt added - Starch: 4g

148 Peanut butter, smooth style, with salt - Starch: 2g

149 Carrots, frozen, cooked, boiled, drained, with salt - Starch: 2g

150 OSCAR MAYER, Wieners (beef franks) [frankfurter, hot dog, hotdog, wiener] 2 g.- Starch